Delay, Denial and Dilution

The Impact of NHS Rationing on Heart Disease and Cancer

IEA Health and Welfare Unit

Choice in Welfare No. 55

Delay, Denial and Dilution:

The Impact of NHS Rationing on Heart Disease and Cancer

David G. Green
Laura Casper

IEA Health and Welfare Unit
London

First published January 2000

IEA Health and Welfare Unit
2 Lord North St
London SW1P 3LB

ISBN 0-255 36459-8
ISSN 1362-9565

Typeset by the IEA Health and Welfare Unit
in New Century Schoolbook

Printed in Great Britain by
St Edmundsbury Press Ltd, Suffolk

Contents

The Authors

David G. Green is the Director of the Health and Welfare Unit at the Institute of Economic Affairs. His books include *Power and Party in an English City*, Allen & Unwin, 1980; *Mutual Aid or Welfare State*, Allen & Unwin, 1984 (with L. Cromwell); *Working-Class Patients and the Medical Establishment*, Temple Smith/ Gower, 1985; *The New Right: The Counter Revolution in Political, Economic and Social Thought*, Wheatsheaf, 1987; *Reinventing Civil Society*, IEA, 1993; *Community Without Politics*, IEA, 1996; *Benefit Dependency*, IEA, 1998; and *An End to Welfare Rights*, IEA, 1999.

He wrote the chapter on 'The Neo-Liberal Perspective' in *The Student's Companion to Social Policy*, Blackwell, 1998.

Laura Casper lives in Wisconsin and is currently studying at Trinity College, Hartford, Connecticut. She worked as a research assistant at the IEA Health and Welfare Unit during the summer of 1999.

Terence Kealey lectures in clinical biochemistry at Cambridge University and is an honorary consultant chemical pathologist at Addenbrooke's Hospital.

Foreword

When in 1987 I toured the university teaching hospital in Aachen, Germany, the Director boasted of his 80 per cent bed occupancy rate. I was surprised. 'But my hospital' I said 'has a 100 per cent bed occupancy rate'.

'You do not understand' he said. 'We have two other big hospitals in Aachen, one has a bed occupancy of 70 per cent and the other of only 60 per cent'.

In Germany, as in most countries of western Europe, there are no waiting lists. Hospitals compete for patients, the professional staff is content, and facilities are modern. In Britain, on the other hand, as Casper and Green demonstrate in this remarkable book, there are waiting lists for the waiting lists. Moreover, neither our doctors nor our nurses are content, and the facilities are poor.

Britain's health service is almost unique. Whereas the countries of western Europe have created systems of health care based on private insurance—but underpinned by the state to ensure that the poor are not neglected—we in Britain use a system modelled on Lenin's dream of universal 'free' provision, and so, in the midst of an expanding and prosperous economy, we in Britain have nurtured an island of Soviet socialism. How well does it work?

Not very well. For decades, the faults of the NHS have been obscured by the general improvements in health that our increased prosperity, improved nutrition and better housing have created, but now that we are prosperous—now that life and death depend on hospitals, doctors and nurses rather than on sewers, agriculture and accommodation—the inadequacies of our health delivery are increasingly being exposed. For years, people have been reluctant to shatter our faith in the 'envy of the world' (an envy so envious that practically nobody has copied us) but in this courageous book Casper and Green have chronicled how poorly the NHS does, in fact, serve the sufferers from the common diseases of our time. Nationalisation works no better in health than in telephones.

Beveridge didn't mean it to be this way. In his famous Report, published in December 1942, he applauded the 'phenomenal growth of voluntary insurance against sickness', and indeed, by

1938, the 1,334 voluntary hospitals of Britain received 59 per cent of their income from patients' fees, paid either directly or via private health insurance organised by institutions such as the British Provident Association.

Beveridge wanted to foster the growth of private medical insurance, and he wanted to restrict the state only to underpinning provision for the poor, but Nye Bevan ('a squalid nuisance' as Winston Churchill once described him) was determined on nationalisation on the Soviet model—and in a classic case of 'crowding out', his universal 'free' provision destroyed private health care for most people.

Of course, UK health care is cheap. We spend less on health care than does any comparable nation, but the cheapness of the NHS is subsidised by the exhaustion and demoralisation of the staff and by the second-rate service it so often provides. It is the cheapness of the miser who knows the price of everything and the value of nothing. And it is a cheapness that demeans patients as supplicants and which hides the medical realities of rationing from them.

Nobody wants to be told to pay more for anything, so the political parties now collude with the people of Britain in pretending they have created a perpetual motion machine—a magical instrument for conjuring truly free health care out of a politician's *fiat*. But the reality is that, after reading this book, people will want better treatment, and they will want to find the money.

Yet, and this has emerged as an iron law of our time, people will not pay higher taxes. They will, however, pay for private goods, so we must now invent a system that lowers the barriers between the private and public sectors, to reward private payers for, in Beveridge's words, 'the duty and pleasure of thrift'.

Put simply, we should copy the German system, but if that policy appears too europhiliac for some, we should copy the Swiss system instead (it's almost identical). Nobody would want to copy the Americans, so let us recognise that health is one area where the Continentals do better than the Anglophones.

In reality, it is the German health care system that is the envy of the world—or it would be, if the world were better informed. Thanks to Casper and Green, it now is.

Terence Kealey

Preface

It is often said that, despite the fact that British expenditure on health care is low by international standards, the British National Health Service produces good medical outcomes. In recent years it has become obvious that there is rationing, but the examples which have received most public attention have affected relatively small groups, such as people suffering from multiple sclerosis or male impotence. The NHS could conceivably be struggling to meet the needs of such special groups without being fundamentally flawed, and a fairer measure of its success would be to look at the impact of the NHS on the killer diseases which affect the most people. We therefore looked at the two main causes of premature death: diseases of the circulatory system (responsible for 40 per cent of premature deaths in men and 30 per cent in women) and cancer (the second biggest killer). Just how well does the NHS do compared with similar countries?

Thanks are due to Laura Casper, who worked at the IEA as a research assistant during the summer of 1999 and produced such good work that I felt it only right to make her a co-author. I have also benefited from the research assistance of Selina Jones, Ben Browning and Katherine Russell, all of whom did a fine job. Ben Browning deserves to be singled out for his invaluable help.

The finished product was much improved by the comments of Lord McColl, Jim Thornton, Robert Whelan and two anonymous referees. Needless to say, any remaining errors, omissions or oversights are entirely my fault.

David G. Green

Introduction

'The NHS is efficient. We spend less on health as a proportion of GDP than many other countries, but the results are just as good.' Such claims are common, but is it true to say that the NHS produces good results for patients? This study examines the impact of the NHS on the two main killer diseases. Among both men and women the biggest cause of death is diseases of the circulatory system, followed by cancer. Among diseases of the circulatory system, we focus on coronary heart disease and stroke. We look at four cancers: breast cancer, the most common cancer for females; lung cancer, the most common for men; colorectal cancer, the second most common fatal malignancy in both sexes combined; and ovarian cancer, the fourth most common amongst women. Does the NHS ration provision for people suffering from these conditions? And if so, does it make any difference to the results for patients?

Until recently, the existence of explicit rationing by the NHS was consistently denied. All decisions were supposed to be clinical rather than financial. There was 'priority setting' but not 'rationing'. Such claims have become increasingly implausible, however, as the number of doctors complaining about rationing has increased.

Just as the outright denial of rationing has become less tenable, so defenders of the NHS have tried to offer a more positive defence. Instead of claiming that all decisions are clinical, they argue that medical rationing is a virtue, so long as decisions are based on legitimate grounds. Typically they assert, not only that rationing exists, but also that it is unavoidable. Invariably they object to medical paternalism and suggest one of four main alternative (sometimes overlapping) rationales.

One group argues that rationing should be given democratic legitimacy, through devices such as opinion surveys and citizen juries.[1] A second group demands evidence-based medicine. Only medical procedures based on scientific evidence should be provided by the NHS. The National Institute for Clinical Excellence (NICE) is a consequence of this line of reasoning. A third group emphasises cost-effectiveness.[2] In practice, they are closely linked to enthusiasts for evidence-based medicine, but not all champions of scientific evidence attach the same weight to cost minimisation. And a fourth group has urged that treatment should be made available according to the quality of life gained by patients. The Quality Adjusted Life Year (QALY) has probably been the most debated of such apparently technical devices.[3]

These enthusiasts for openness and explicit rationing have in their turn come under strong criticism by writers such as David Hunter[4] and Rudolf Klein,[5] who have tended to debunk 'rational rationing'. The purpose of the present study, however, is not to enter into that debate, but to form a clearer view about the extent of rationing on the two biggest causes of death in the UK, diseases of the circulatory system and cancer.

Before going any further it may be advisable to clarify what we mean by rationing. It is inevitable that words will take on alternative meanings in different contexts, but it is rather important that any one word should mean the same thing during the course of any single argument. We follow Rudolf Klein in distinguishing between priority setting and rationing.[6] If a service is financed from taxes, the government will inevitably be guided by priorities when it apportions some of the national budget to the NHS or elements within it. We do not call this process rationing, but when individual doctors, working within their assigned budgets, make decisions about the treatment of individual patients, then we speak of rationing.

Measures of Rationing: Denial, Delay and Dilution

One example which has received attention in the press and specialist journals is the *denial* of cancer care, so much so that the Prime Minister himself became involved. The most authoritative estimate has been made by Professor Sikora, head of the WHO cancer programme, who calculated that there could be as many as

25,000 unnecessary deaths in the UK every year because of under-provision. We can also compare the rate at which care is denied to people suffering from kidney failure. A recent survey of renal specialists in Canada, the US and the UK found that 12 per cent of UK specialists said they had refused treatment to patients because of limited resources. The rate of provision between the three countries varied substantially. In 1992, 65 patients per million population (pmp) were accepted for dialysis in the UK, compared with 98 pmp in Canada and 212 pmp in the US.[7] According to another study, by 1995 the figure for England was 82 pmp, significantly less than the rate in comparable European countries, where acceptance rates of over 100 pmp were common. The authors estimated that the rate in England should exceed 100 pmp to meet established need.[8]

Often treatment is not withheld altogether, but it is *delayed*, sometimes with the result that the patient's condition worsens. There are measures of delay, not least the waiting lists, although their impact on outcomes is not always clear cut. *The National Survey of NHS Patients*, published by the Department of Health, is also a useful guide. It found that one in ten patients were seen by a specialist on the same day as they were referred by their GP. About 50 per cent had to wait over a month and 20 per cent more than three months. Over one in three of those waiting said that their condition had got worse while they were waiting and 14 per cent claimed to be 'in a lot of pain'. Over 50 per cent reported that their condition limited their daily activities and ability to work and, not surprisingly, of the men of working age (16-64), half thought they should have been seen sooner.[9]

The waiting list has been the focus of much political attention since the Government's election pledge to cut it. Its efforts have, however, led to continuing claims that it was 'fiddling' the figures. One ploy used by some hospitals to avoid going over the 18-months threshold is to call in patients who have been waiting for *nearly* 18 months for a check-up. If they are put back on the waiting list the clock starts ticking from zero, thus concealing the real waiting time. Moreover, the Government was forced in the summer of 1999 to acknowledge that its reduction in the waiting list had been achieved by increasing the time it took to see a consultant in the first place. There was now a 'waiting list for the waiting list'.

Care may also be *diluted* by not providing the optimal treatment. This often happens when new but expensive remedies become available. Again, demonstrating the impact of diluted care on outcomes is not easy and systematic evidence is not readily available. Moreover, there is invariably no clear-cut agreement among doctors about which treatments are 'appropriate' or 'optimal'. We are not, however, wholly unable to judge between rival treatments. A variety of organisations have produced clinical guidelines, protocols and recommendations which enjoy wide respect, either in the UK or overseas. If a given doctor or hospital or system (such as the NHS) falls short of a well-respected clinical guideline this constitutes at least *prima facie* evidence of dilution and calls for further investigation. Among the official organisations laying down benchmarks in the UK are the Clinical Standards Advisory Group[10] and the Standing Medical Advisory Committee,[11] and such work is to be stepped up through the Commission for Health Improvement and the National Service Frameworks.

1

Diseases of the Circulatory System

Over 40 per cent of all deaths are the result of cardiovascular disease (CVD). The two main forms of CVD are coronary heart disease (including heart attacks and angina) and cerebrovascular disease (stroke). In 1996 just over half of all deaths from CVD were from coronary heart disease and about a quarter from stroke.[1] However, we must all die of something and the more relevant figure is for 'premature' deaths, namely those occurring before age 75. In 1996 cardiovascular disease was responsible for over 40 per cent of premature deaths in men and 30 per cent in women.[2]

The Government admits that the UK record is unsatisfactory. After allowing for the different age structure of each country, *Saving Lives: Our Healthier Nation* compares death rates from circulatory disease for persons aged under 65 throughout the European Union. Out of the 15 countries studied, the UK was thirteenth.[3]

Coronary Heart Disease

Coronary heart disease (CHD) is the most common cause of premature (under the age of 75) death in the UK, accounting for 28 per cent of premature deaths in men and 17 per cent in women in 1996—nearly 60,000 premature deaths in total.[4]

For some years now UK governments have officially sought to reduce deaths from coronary heart disease,[5] but CHD death rates remain among the highest in the world. The former communist countries tend to be the worst. As Figure 1 shows, the rate for men aged 35-74 in Latvia in 1994 was 919 per 100,000 population (age-standardised). In the Russian Federation it was 812 per 100,000; in Estonia, 744; Lithuania, 663; and Bulgaria, 352. Compared only with OECD countries the UK record is also poor (Figure 2).

Figure 1
Coronary Heart Disease Death Rates for Men Aged 35-74 per 100,000 Population (1993 or 1994) Selected Countries

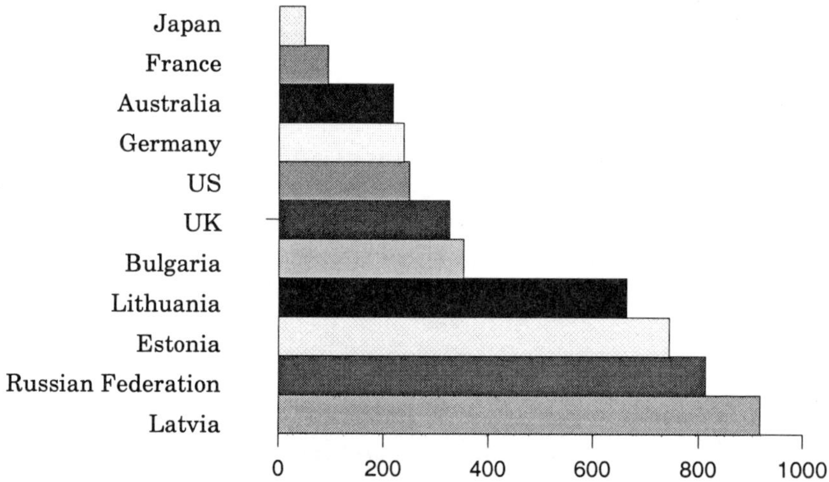

Source: *Coronary Heart Disease Statistics*, British Heart Foundation, 1998, p. 19.

Western countries and Japan tend to have lower rates. Japan's figure is 49 per 100,000; France, 94; Canada, 212; Australia, 217; Germany, 237; and the US, 248 (in 1993). In the UK the rate of 325 per 100,000 in 1994 is closer to the Bulgarian figure. Death rates from CHD have been falling in the UK, but not as rapidly as in some other countries like Australia, Sweden and the US. Between 1983 and 1993 the death rate for men in the UK fell by 30 per cent, compared with 43 per cent in Australia, 41 per cent in Sweden and 34 per cent in the USA.[6]

However, the *Health Survey for England* and the *General Household Survey* suggest that while death from CHD is falling, the incidence of *ill-health* due to CHD is not falling and may in fact be rising. Drawing on a variety of sources, the British Heart Foundation (BHF) estimates that approximately 300,000 people in the UK have a heart attack each year and that about 1.4 million people have angina.[7]

Figure 2
Ischaemic Heart Disease,
Deaths Per 100,000 Population, 1995

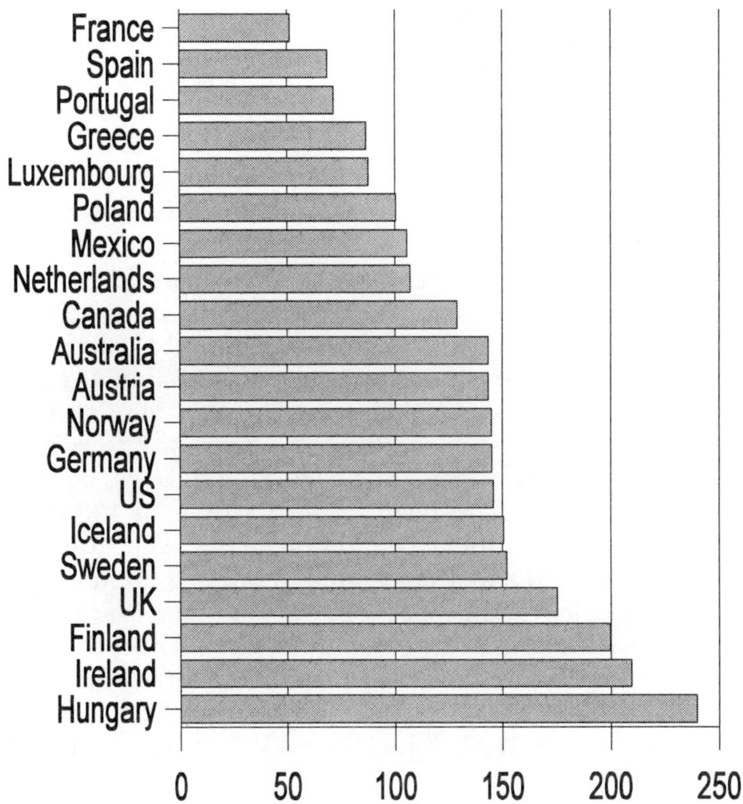

Source: OECD Health Data 1999 (CD)

Heart disease has major economic consequences as well as human costs. CHD alone cost the healthcare system about £1.6 billion in 1996, with about 55 per cent going to hospital care and

32 per cent on the cost of drugs. Only about one per cent of such costs were spent on the prevention of CHD. The British Heart Foundation has estimated the total impact of CHD on the UK economy to be about £10 billion a year.[8]

The Adequacy of CHD Treatment

CHD leads to the obstruction of the blood flow through the coronary arteries to the heart muscle, due to fatty deposits and associated blood clots. An inadequate supply of oxygen-enriched blood to the heart can damage the heart muscle leading to heart pain (angina) or to a heart attack (myocardial infarction) that may be fatal. CHD is influenced by several factors, not all of which can be altered. The genetic risk cannot be changed by medical intervention but cigarette smoking, high blood cholesterol levels, raised blood pressure, obesity and lack of exercise can all be modified by lifestyle choices and/or medical treatment.

The most common treatment is to take drugs, although angina can also be treated surgically, in the form of coronary artery bypass grafts (CABGs) or angioplasty.[9] CABGs usually involve grafting veins or arteries (taken from the leg) from the aorta (a major artery that takes blood from the heart to the rest of the body) to the coronary artery, thus bypassing the obstructed area. Government targets have been set for CABGs. In 1986 the UK target was 300 per million population (pmp). The number had risen between 1978 and 1985 from 57 pmp to 225 pmp in 1987. The *Health of the Nation* report of 1991 conceded that the target of 300 pmp was 'significantly below most targets adopted by other countries',[10] and noted that even this inadequate target had not been achieved. In 1990 the rate was only 278 pmp (15,967 operations) but by 1996 it had increased to 412 pmp (24,238 operations).[11] At the time, the British Cardiac Society target was 600 per million population.[12]

The UK rate compares very unfavourably with the US, where 598,000 CABGs were performed in 1996, at a rate of 2,255 per million population.[13] The rate for Australia was about 870 pmp; Canada, 582 pmp and Sweden, 736 pmp.[14]

Not only is the overall rate low, the Department of Health also concedes that there are large variations between different parts of the country. Adjusting for age, the lowest figure was for the Nottingham Health Authority where only 40 bypass operations and angioplasties per million population were carried out. The highest rate was found in Brent and Harrow with 1,400 per million.[15] These local disparities had been identified by the Audit Commission report of 1995, which urged health authorities with rates below 300 pmp to give priority to increasing supply.[16] Progress has been very slow.

The consequences are serious. A study of Papworth Hospital found that deaths occur while patients are on waiting lists for CABGs. Moreover, for every one death on the waiting list there were between two and three adverse cardiac events. The authors concluded that the high mortality and complication rates while waiting were because resource limits meant that patients tended to be put on waiting lists only when their condition had become urgent. They concluded that 'many UK patients are referred and investigated at a critical stage in their disease and are therefore at high risk at the time of invasive intervention'. This tendency suggested to the authors that the surgical treatment of coronary heart disease in the UK was 'more a form of crisis management than planned care'.[17]

Moreover, because of the prevalence of rationing, doctors have fallen into the habit of withholding treatment on non-clinical grounds. In their 1993 report,[18] the Clinical Standards Advisory Group drew attention to the lack of clear criteria for giving priority to patients waiting for coronary artery bypass surgery. In response to this report, a regional workshop sponsored by the Northern Ireland Clinical Resource Efficiency Support Team convened in the spring of 1996 to gain a better understanding of the criteria used by doctors to assign priority to particular patients. Many doctors made judgements about the urgency of the patient's condition, that is they formed a view about how quickly each patient should be treated in order to achieve a given medical outcome. However, the study also found that demographic and lifestyle characteristics–such as smoking, age, gender and body weight–often influenced doctors' judgements on priority independently of their beliefs about the probable effectiveness of surgery.[19] These findings are consistent with the long-standing practice of discriminating against elderly patients[20] because they have 'had a good innings', and with the acknowledged practice of discriminating against smokers, which is publicly defended by some doctors.[21]

High Blood Pressure

The two main risk factors for CHD which are susceptible to medical intervention are high blood pressure and the blood cholesterol level. (Smoking is a personal choice and obesity is controllable in most cases through changes in diet and exercise.) How effectively is high blood pressure being dealt with by the NHS? High blood pressure or hypertension is usually a symptomless condition which increases the risk of stroke, heart failure, heart attack and kidney failure. It is the most important risk factor for stroke. Because there are no symptoms in the majority of cases, high blood pressure often goes undetected.

When blood pressure is measured two figures are recorded: the highest occurs when the heart contracts (systolic); and the lowest when the heart relaxes between beats (diastolic). Blood pressure is usually written with the higher number first, for example 160/95 mmHg. The mean systolic blood pressure for men in England is about 139 mmHg and for women 134mmHg. The British Heart Foundation defines individuals as hypertensive if their systolic blood pressure is more than 160 mmHg and their diastolic blood pressure is more than 95 mmHg.[22] There is no clear medical consensus about the point at which blood pressure is high enough to warrant intervention, although it is accepted that the higher the blood pressure the greater the risk.

Treatment involves a combination of lifestyle changes and drug therapies.[23] Lifestyle changes generally come first. People who are overweight are strongly advised to lose weight and smokers to give up. Changes in diet, especially for those with high blood cholesterol levels or complications such as diabetes, are also strongly recommended. Reducing sodium and salt intake, without reducing the consumption of calcium, magnesium or potassium, and reducing alcohol intake are also highly beneficial.

Medically, a common first step is a thiazide diuretic. This group of drugs works by helping the kidneys to eliminate salt and water, which decreases fluid in the body thus lowering blood pressure. Thiazide diuretics also cause blood vessels to dilate, increasing their capacity and lowering blood pressure.

Another approach is to block some of the body's natural defence mechanisms. Under stress, or in moments of danger, the sympathetic nervous system temporarily increases blood pressure to cope with threats and releases hormones, such as adrenalin, which stimulate the heart and blood vessels. Adrenergic blockers, the most common of which are the beta-blockers, reduce the effects of the sympathetic nervous system.

A third approach is to use angiotensin converting enzyme (ACE) inhibitors, which lower blood pressure by dilating the arteries.[24]

It is now widely acknowledged that ACE inhibitors are effective and safe remedies when used appropriately. For example, it is the recommendation of the North of England ACE-inhibitor Guideline Development Group that 'all patients with symptomatic heart failure and evidence of impaired left ventricular function' as well as those with 'a recent myocardial infarction' and evidence of left ventricular dysfunction should be treated with an ACE inhibitor.[25] The great majority of adults with heart failure have left ventricular dysfunction. However, a study carried out by the group found that only 20-30 per cent of patients with heart failure were being prescribed an ACE inhibitor.[26]

This finding is similar to those of two Scottish studies. The first, by the Scotland Health Purchasing Information Centre, found that an ACE inhibitor was being prescribed for only around one-third of patients diagnosed with heart failure in general practice in Scotland and that, even when prescribed, patients often received sub-optimal doses.[27] The second study looked at patients in the Grampian region and found that, under the management of general practitioners, less than half the patients diagnosed with heart failure took ACE inhibitors. Indeed, less than one-third of patients with a recent myocardial infarction took beta blockers, despite the fact that their use has achieved mortality reductions of 20 per cent following heart attack.[28]

These practices compare badly with those prevalent overseas. One study of US practice between 1986 and 1994 examined the use of ACE inhibitors in combination with a diuretic and digitalis. Since 1987 it had been widely accepted that ACE inhibitors improved survival for patients with heart failure and symptomatic left ventricular dysfunction. Of patients who were hospitalised for heart failure in 1986 and 1987, 43 per cent were prescribed an ACE inhibitor, whereas of those hospitalised in 1992 and 1993, 71 per cent were prescribed an ACE inhibitor.[29]

Not only is there evidence of under-use of valuable therapies, there is also evidence of inadequate diagnosis. There are some less common causes of heart failure, such as aortic valve obstruction, where ACE inhibitors are unhelpful or harmful, and therefore accurate diagnosis is essential. Diagnosis is greatly aided by the ultrasound technique known as echocardiography, which can produce images of the heart and show how well the muscle is contracting. It can usually establish the cause, and confirm the presence of heart failure and thus allow the correct use of drugs.[30]

However, a study of the NHS in Scotland showed that only 30 per cent of heart failure patients in general practice were given echocardiography scans despite evidence from areas where echocardiography was freely available that 'important changes in treatment' were required in 69 per cent of patients referred.[31] Moreover, echocardiography was not expensive—about £45 per scan in Glasgow. The Scotland Health Purchasing Information Centre (SHPIC) recommended provision of a one-stop cardiology service, but in deference to the NHS tradition of rationing, even though such a service would be cheap and cost-effective, the group recommended a second-best option of a GP echocardiography service in the hope of reducing by about two-thirds the cases requiring referral to a hospital.[32]

A second study by the North of England ACE-inhibitor Guideline Development Group drew similar conclusions. It found that most patients who were investigated for heart failure had a chest X-ray and electrocardiogram, while only a third had echocardiography. Diagnosis by clinical assessment had been estimated to be correct in only about half of cases when confirmed by echocardiography.[33] It recommended that diagnosis should be based on either echocardiography or radionuclide measurement.[34]

To sum up: the NHS does not have a very good record of providing these tried and tested remedies. According to the British Heart Foundation, based on the 1996 Health Survey for England, over four out of ten men and over one in three women with hypertension were not receiving treatment and, of those that are treated, about a third remain hypertensive.[35] Even the Government has acknowledged that fewer than half of people with high blood pressure are treated successfully. In 1997, 42 per cent of people with hypertension were being treated successfully, 21 per cent were being treated inadequately and 37 per cent were not being treated at all.[36]

Cholesterol

A second CHD risk factor is the blood cholesterol level. According to the British Heart Foundation, lowering blood cholesterol levels by one per cent reduces the risk of CHD by about two to three per cent.[37]

Cholesterol is a fatty substance which can be found in several forms in the human body. When bound to proteins it forms lipoprotein. Cholesterol and other fatty blood components are often called 'blood lipids' and can be divided into two groups: low-density lipoprotein (LDL) cholesterol and high-density lipoprotein (HDL) cholesterol. High levels of LDL cholesterol and *low* levels of HDL cholesterol are associated with an increased risk of CHD.

A new class of cholesterol-lowering drugs, the statins (HMG CoA reductase inhibitors), are able to reduce LDL cholesterol levels by more than 20 per cent.[38] The first trial to show that CHD patients treated with lipid-lowering drugs gained a survival advantage was the Scandinavian trial, published in November 1994.[39] A Scottish trial confirmed this result[40] and subsequently a total of 22 published randomised controlled trials of cholesterol lowering with statins have been pooled. Overall, they show that statins reduce the risk of CHD mortality by about 25 per cent and that statin treatment in older people is just as effective as in middle-aged adults.[41]

These findings have led to increased expenditure on statin drugs. In 1993 expenditure was over £20m and by 1997 it had risen to over £113m.[42] Enthusiasts for cost-effectiveness have also found in favour of statins. The net cost per life-year gained with statins of around £7,000, though quite high, compares favourably with other interventions currently provided by the NHS.[43]

To what extent has the NHS acted on the known evidence? The British Cardiac Society conducted a national sample survey to assess the adequacy of heart disease treatment. It found that 'the recording and management of risk factors—lifestyle, blood pressure, cholesterol, glucose—and the use of prophylactic drug treatment were less than optimal'. For example, according to the British Hyperlipidaemia Association's (BHA) guidelines, most of the patients in the survey should have been attempting to lower their LDL cholesterol either by dietary change or drug treatment. Of the minority of patients on lipid lowering treatment, over half were not 'adequately controlled' according to the BHA guidelines.[44]

Another study of the prescribing of lipid lowering drugs in the South East Thames Region found dramatic variations. Within a single health authority, prescribing varied by 60-fold between practices, and across the region the variation was 98-fold.[45] A Scottish study concluded that 'lipid management' was 'largely neglected', despite the existence of local guidelines advocating cholesterol lowering for patients with CHD. The blood pressure of 93 per cent of patients in the survey had been measured in the previous three years, whereas their blood cholesterol level had been checked in only 26 per cent of cases during the same period.[46]

Is the erratic provision the result of rationing or is it bad clinical practice? Recent discussion in the medical journals provides some insights. In August 1997, the Standing Medical Advisory Committee (SMAC) issued advice to health authorities and GPs on the use of statins. It recommended that anyone with a three per cent annual risk of a heart attack should be treated.[47] This meant that about 3.4 per cent of those aged 35-69 in England were eligible for statins in addition to those who had already experienced a CHD event.[48] However, Nick Freemantle, Senior Research Fellow at the Centre for Health Economics, subsequently attacked the modest SMAC guidelines in an editorial in the *British Medical Journal* as financially unsustainable. He pointed out that the SMAC guidelines would mean that 8.2 per cent of the population of those aged 35-69 would have to be treated to fulfil all the priorities. In the Warwickshire Health Authority alone, adhering to the SMAC guidelines would involve treating about 17,000 patients. The cost in Warwickshire would be about £8m, representing 20 per cent of its drug budget.[49] Such concerns have not been confined to Warwickshire, and the result has been substantial under-use of statins. As the 1999 report of the Audit Commission remarked, there was evidence that drug therapies for preventing CHD 'were not being used as much as they usefully could be'.[50]

Heart Attacks

The Audit Commission in 1995 suggested some performance indicators for patients arriving at a hospital with chest pain and/or other symptoms of a heart attack. The ideal to aim for would be to carry out an electrocardiogram (ECG) within 15 minutes of arrival and, when a myocardial infarction is suspected, to administer thrombolytic therapy within 30 minutes of arrival (often called the door-to-needle time).[51] These recommendations are often not achieved. Moreover, one survey found that a significant minority of key hospital managers did not even know what their achievements were. A survey of 500 trust chairmen, chief executives, medical directors and chief nurses carried out by the *Health Service Journal* and the Health Quality Service asked respondents to give a 'yes' or 'no' response to the following statement: 'At least 80 per cent of A&E patients with chest pains had a care plan initiated within 30 minutes of arrival.' Only 60 per cent of chairmen answered 'Yes', compared with 47 per cent of chief executives, 57 per cent of medical directors and 70 per cent of chief nurses. The remainder typically answered 'Don't know' rather than 'No'.[52]

Cardiac rehabilitation after heart attack can also significantly improve the quality of life and reduce mortality. The most appropriate forms of rehabilitation combine exercise with psychological and educational services. Evidence from three meta-analyses involving over 4,000 patients who had suffered a heart attack suggests that cardiac mortality can be reduced by 20-25 per cent. However, many patients who might benefit do not receive rehabilitation under the NHS. The York Centre for Reviews and Dissemination found that, despite increases in rehabilitation in recent years, service provision in 1998 failed to meet national guidelines for cardiac rehabilitation. Moreover, there were wide variations in the standard of provision, reflected in staffing costs which ranged from about £10,000 per year to £62,000 per year.[53]

Stroke

Stroke is the nation's third biggest killer and largest single cause of severe disability.[54] The *Health Survey for England 1996* found that 1.8 per cent of men and 1.6 per cent of women reported a history of stroke and that 8.6 per cent of men over the age of 75 and 7.5 per cent of women over 75 reported a history of stroke.[55] However, the *Health Survey for England* relies on self-reporting, and a more reliable estimate has been made by Geddes and her colleagues based on a survey of the North Yorkshire Health Authority. The team estimated that 4.7 per cent of people aged 55 or more had survived a stroke: 80 per cent had suffered a single stroke, 13 per cent, two strokes and seven per cent, three or more. Some 23 per cent reported a full recovery and the remainder experienced subsequent impairments. The most prevalent were cognitive (33 per cent), problems with the right limb (33 per cent), the left limb (27 per cent) and speech (27 per cent). Some 55 per cent said they needed help to fulfil one or more of ten 'activities of daily living'. Overall the study estimated the prevalence of stroke in the whole population to be 1.47 per cent, more than double the estimate normally used by health authorities (0.6 per cent). They estimated that 1.13 per cent of people had impairments and that 0.62 per cent were dependent as a result of their stroke.[56]

Using data from the Geddes survey, the Stroke Association has estimated that 82,000 people aged 55-64 have a history of stroke. Overall, it thought that 764,000 people of all ages in the UK had a history of stroke, of which some 53,000 had severe disabilities as a consequence.[57]

Stroke care costs are considerable. At present, expenditure on stroke care is concentrated on the immediate episode of in-patient treatment and not on long-term care. Overall, the costs of stroke care were £2.3 billion in England in 1995-96. This amounts to 5.8 per cent of NHS and social services expenditure. The cost of longer-term care for surviving stroke patients is also high and likely to rise further as a result of demographic change.[58]

Stroke care already has a strong evidence base. Over the last two decades a number of small, randomised controlled trials of specialised stroke units have been conducted. They found that stroke units reduce mortality and disability compared with management in acute general wards. No other treatment for stroke has demonstrated such large benefits.

For example, a study published in 1994 compared a stroke unit and a general ward. Patients within the stroke unit recovered more quickly as determined by their 'activities of daily living' scores. Patients were also discharged more rapidly from the stroke unit. About half were discharged from the stroke unit in about six weeks compared with over 12 weeks in the general ward. In the stroke unit, all patients were discharged after 12 weeks, whereas it took 32 weeks in the general ward.[59]

In 1993 Peter Langhorne and his colleagues assessed the conclusions that could be drawn from ten randomised clinical trials then available for study. They compared a stroke unit with alternatives such as a general hospital ward. By a stroke unit they meant a multi-disciplinary team of specialists, which could be geographically based or mobile. They found that the management of patients in a stroke unit was associated with lower mortality after 17 weeks and after 12 months. After 12 months, the reduction in mortality was 21 per cent, or 25 per cent if the trials based on informal randomisation were excluded. The study also found evidence that patients treated in units had an improved ability to function.[60]

Special stroke units not only reduce mortality but also reduce the length of hospital stays. The Stroke Unit Trialists Collaboration studied 11 trials comparing a dedicated stroke unit with a general medical ward; six trials comparing mixed assessment/rehabilitation units with a general medical ward; and four trials comparing a mixed assessment/rehabilitation unit with a dedicated unit. Dedicated units dealt with stroke cases only. Mixed assessment/rehabilitation units were either a ward or a team with an interest and expertise in the assessment and rehabilitation of disabling illness but not exclusive to stroke. The rate of death after one year was found to be 20.9 per cent for stroke units and 25.4 per cent for alternatives. The proportion of patients unable to live at home was 40.1 per cent for stroke units and 47.2 per cent for the alternatives. Benefits did not depend on increased hospitals stays and may even have reduced them. The team concluded that stroke unit care was unlikely to be more expensive than conventional care in a general ward and may be less costly.[61]

However, despite clear evidence that stroke units are effective, they are under-used. The most systematic evidence comes from the 1998 Stroke Association survey. It carried out two national surveys: one covering all consultants in the UK responsible for the care of stroke patients; and one covering all health authorities and boards in the UK. The findings were disturbing. The earlier Stroke Association survey of 1992/93 had found that under half of consultants had access to a stroke unit. Despite the appeal of the Stroke Association for the collection of information, in 1999 there was still no national information about the number of stroke units, the treatment policies they followed, or the number of patients treated by them.

Nevertheless, the 1998 survey found that about 75 per cent of consultants had access to 'some form of specialist stroke service', either a defined unit with beds or an interdisciplinary team. However, of those with access to a specialist service, in 46 per cent of cases it was to a rehabilitation unit. Acute-only units were available to 17 per cent of consultants and combined acute/rehabilitation units to 16 per cent.[62]

Consultants were said to be 'fairly happy' with their access, but a significant minority reported inadequate access: 18 per cent had inadequate access to acute stroke units; 20 per cent to rehabilitation units; 25 per cent to acute/rehabilitation units; and 13 per cent to a stroke team.

In practice, however, only one-third of consultants said that patients were usually managed by a stroke unit team or in a stroke unit. Moreover, there were significant regional variations and, in the worst cases of the West Midlands and the North West,

40 per cent of consultants did not manage their patients in stroke units or teams.[63]

Despite an overall improvement in access since 1992/93, the 1998 survey found wide and unacceptable variations around the country in the chances of being managed in an organised stroke service. Consultants from England (29 per cent) and Wales (21 per cent) had poorer access to acute stroke unit care than those from Scotland (41 per cent) or Northern Ireland (52 per cent). Patients in Northern Ireland had the best chance of being admitted or transferred to a stroke unit, followed by Scotland, Trent, Wales and London. Those admitted to hospitals in Wales, Scotland or Northern Ireland were approximately twice as likely to be cared for in a stroke unit as those admitted to English hospitals.[64]

Of those consultants who treated stroke, only 3 per cent were specialists in stroke medicine. The others were specialists in general medicine (55 per cent), geriatric medicine (27 per cent) and neurology (6 per cent). Most were part of a team, but the survey found that many consultants felt the time available for their stroke patients was either 'fairly or very inadequate'.[65]

At the time of the survey it was estimated that on any single day there would be about 10,500 stroke patients in UK hospital beds. On the day of the survey about 52 per cent were managed by an 'organised stroke service'. That is, nearly half were deprived of the established advantages of a stroke unit, namely a substantially reduced risk of death or severe disability. The Stroke Association calculated that, of the estimated 116,000 acute stroke admissions in a year, about 55,000 were not managed in a stroke unit, which would have reduced the chances of death or being institutionalised by 25 per cent. The Stroke Association estimated that this meant there were between 4,500 and 7,000 avoidable deaths and institutional placements each year. Or, counting only deaths, between 2,000 and 3,000 avoidable deaths per year. All told, the Stroke Association concluded that only about half of all stroke patients were receiving 'optimal specialist stroke care'.[66]

The Stroke Association also found that other treatment techniques of proven efficacy were not being applied. There was evidence that some consultants were not well informed about the benefits of some drug treatments, including even aspirin and heparin, which had been the subject of two major international trials the year before the survey. When patients were treated in the community, the Stroke Association found that fewer than half of the patients who would benefit from taking aspirin were in fact taking it. And, even following hospital discharge, only 80 per cent were taking it.[67]

2

Cancer

In *Saving Lives: Our Healthier Nation* the Government reports that overall death rates from cancer in England for people under 65 are slightly better than the EU average, but goes on to say that this figure conceals some important differences. The UK rate of death from breast cancer is amongst the worst in Europe, twelfth out of 15, and for cervical cancer the UK is thirteenth out of 15.[1] The report makes the further admission that the chances of surviving are poorer in the UK than in some other countries and goes on to concede that 'part of the difference may reflect the fact that there are cancer services in other countries which are better than we are in this country at treating cancer'. This admission is then followed by a further confession. People in 'more deprived areas', it says, 'tend to have lower survival rates'.[2]

The Eurocare II study, based on over 3.4 million cancer records in 17 countries, allows us to compare survival rates in England and Scotland with those for other European countries.[3] It showed that in England and Scotland the five-year survival rate from 1985 to 1989 was below the European average for both men and women suffering cancer of the colon and rectum,[4] lung,[5] and breast.[6] The gap was often substantial. For instance, five years after treatment, the chances of survival for men with colorectal cancer were 59 per cent in the Netherlands compared with 41 per cent in England and Scotland. In France men with lung cancer had a 40 per cent chance of being alive five years after treatment, compared with 23 per cent in England.

Since the report of the Expert Advisory Group on Cancer (Calman-Hine) in 1995[7] more attention has been devoted to deficiencies in cancer care. However, despite the widespread criticism, inadequacies remain. According to WHO cancer programme director and NHS consultant, Professor Karol Sikora, no major resources have been allocated to setting up specialist teams, as recommended by Calman-Hine, and the UK has fewer oncologists per patient than comparable European countries. A Royal College of Radiologists' survey found that the workload of UK oncologists was far higher than in similar European countries. Some UK consultants were seeing over 1,000 new patients a year. The average was 550 a year, compared with 250 in France and Germany. To match German and French figures would require the number of UK consultants to be doubled.[8]

The shortage of specialists means, not only the denial of treatment, but also delays even in emergencies. For instance, metastatic malignant spinal cord compression is a major cause of morbidity in patients with cancer and often means that a previously-functioning patient becomes bedridden or confined to hospital for the rest of his or her life.

D.J. Husband, consultant in clinical oncology in Bebington, carried out a study of 301 patients referred to the Clatterbridge Centre for Oncology for treatment of a first episode of malignant spinal cord compression during a three-year period. It is widely accepted that malignant spinal cord compression is a medical or surgical emergency, requiring urgent diagnosis and treatment because dely can result in irreversible paralysis or loss of bladder function.

However, the study found that delay in the diagnosis and treatment of malignant spinal cord compression remained a common problem and resulted in preventable deterioration in neurological function before treatment in most patients. It is reasonable to expect referral and treatment of this condition in less than 24 hours but the study found that this target was not achieved for 70 per cent of patients at general practitioner stage, 79 per cent at the district general hospital stage, and 33 per cent at the treatment unit stage. Delays of more than seven days occurred in 33 per cent of patients at the general practitioner stage, 34 per cent at the district general hospital stage and six per cent at the treatment unit stage. Failure to diagnose spinal cord compression and failure to investigate, refer, and treat sufficiently urgently were the main causes of delay and the consequent functional deterioration.[9]

The Calman-Hine report advocated an improved network of care based on some 30 specialist cancer centres, each linked to 10-12 cancer units. In the year after the Calman-Hine report, Professor Richards and colleagues[10] conducted a survey based on 12 trusts providing for 24 million people. The study looked at current activity levels, changes in activity over time, and facilities for cancer care. They found that the recommendations of the Calman-Hine report had not been implemented. Five out of the twelve centres did not provide a full haemato-oncology service and the same number did not employ specialists in palliative medicine. Furthermore, considerable inequalities were evident in the provision of high technology equipment, the referral rate and the provision of cancer beds between the centres.[11] Three years later, in 1999, Professor Karol Sikora described the implementation of Calman-Hine as a 'saga of under-resourcing and bureaucratic muddle'. Whole forests had been felled, he said, to generate the paper consumed by reports, strategic analyses and focus groups, but progress had been inadequate. A major problem had been 'the lack of new resources to implement change'.[12]

If the UK were as effective in treating each cancer as the best in Europe, argued Professor Sikora, it could save up to 25,000 lives a year. And if it merely hit the average, this figure would be 10,000 lives.[13] He conceded that there had been some improvements, but because the Calman-Hine report had not been accompanied by any promise of new funding, any improvements implied a reduction in other services. He thought that the limited improvements following Calman-Hine had been at the expense of patients with cardiovascular disease, diabetes and the chronic problems of old age.[14]

The Main Kinds of Cancer

Lung Cancer

Surgical resection is the recognised treatment of choice for patients with stage I or II non-small cell lung cancer. In the UK surgical resection rates have remained at about 10 per cent, whereas in the USA one survey reported a rate of 28 per cent and in Europe rates have been found to be higher still. In reality, many UK patients with operable tumours have been denied the chance of curative surgery.[15]

Figure 3

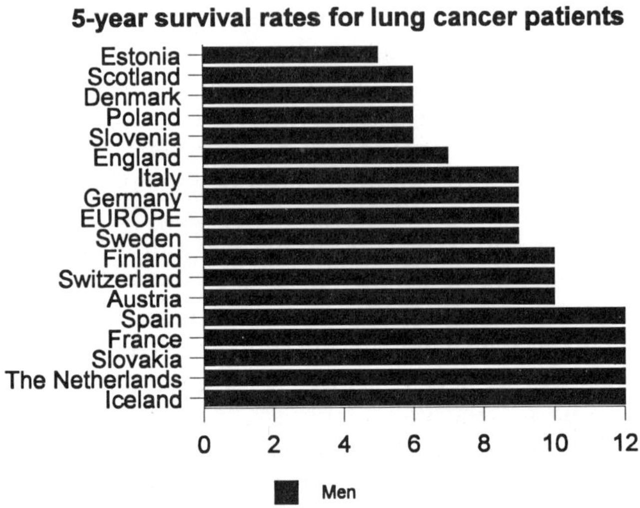

Figure 4

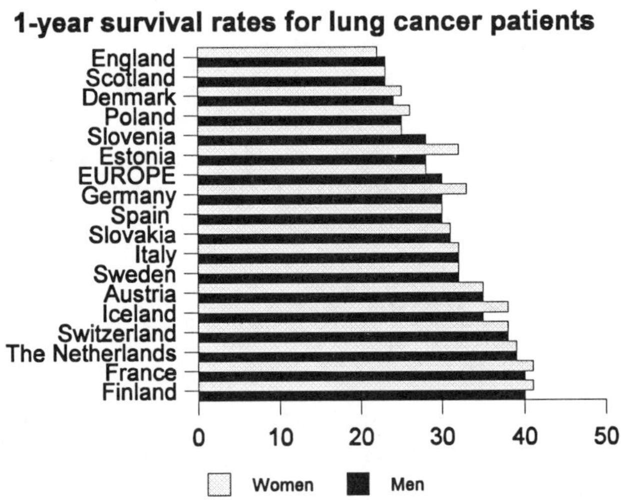

Note: All rates are relative and age-standardised. They reflect findings from the Eurocare II study for 1985-1989.

The one-year survival rates in England and Scotland were not only below the European average, but the absolute lowest out of the 17 countries–which included Estonia, Slovakia, Slovenia and the other 14 countries in the Eurocare II study (see Figure 4). The five-year survival rates for England and Scotland were also well below the European average but were not the absolute lowest. Estonia had a five per cent survival rate for men compared with Scotland's six per cent and England's seven per cent (see Figure 3). The Eurocare II authors believed that the lower survival rates for patients with lung cancer in England and Scotland were partly explained by restricted access to specialised care.[16]

Hilary Pickles, Director of Public Health in Hillingdon, has argued that lung cancer is often given low priority because it is seen as 'self-inflicted'. Pickles further argued that only so much can be done within existing resources and that the outlook for lung cancer compared with alternatives such as care of the elderly, asthma, breast cancer and cardiothoracic surgery was bleak.[17]

Breast Cancer

Each year around 30,000 new cases of breast cancer are diagnosed in the UK and around 15,000 die from the disease. The Eurocare study, based on 30 cancer registries in 12 countries between 1978 and 1985, found relatively low survival for UK women with breast cancer. England and Scotland, along with Spain, Estonia and Poland, had the lowest rates of breast cancer survival.[18] The Eurocare II study from 1985 to 1989, based on 42 registries in 17 countries, found that Scotland, England and Slovenia had one-year survival some 3-4 per cent below the average, and five-year survival 6-9 per cent below average (see Figure 5).[19]

How can these differences be explained? The Eurocare authors concluded that low survival in the UK may be attributed to poor compliance on the part of health authorities and doctors with consensus treatment guidelines as well as greater variations in treatment.[20]

There is no evidence that breast cancer in UK women differs in histology or grade from that in similar countries. Nor is there evidence that women in the UK who have symptomatic breast disease delay any longer in seeking diagnosis.[21] Consequently, according to Professor Richards of Guys and St Thomas', the chief reason for poor UK results is that a significant number of women who are diagnosed with breast cancer receive 'sub-optimal care'.[22] A study of women aged under 50 in the South East Thames Region by Professor Richards found that the treatments provided were 'frequently at variance' with well-respected guidelines.[23]

Figure 5

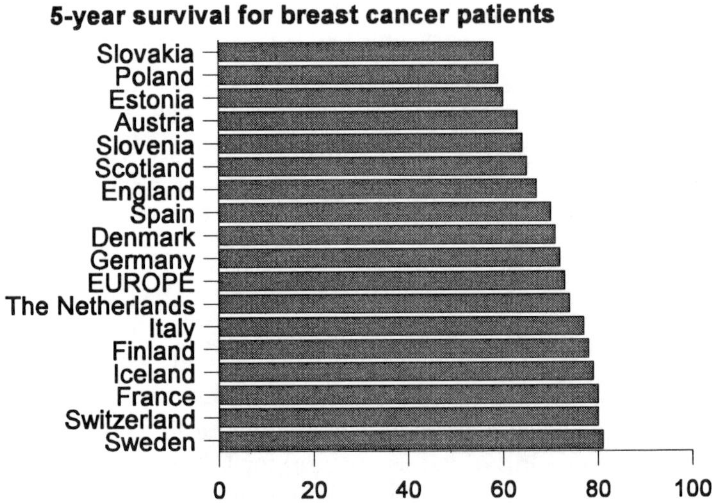

Note: Rates are age standardised and relative. 1985-1989 Eurocare II

A study by C.J. Twelves and colleagues found that, although geographical variations in the selection of patients for surgery account for some of the differences in survival, the health authority in which the patient was first treated had an effect on the outcome. In fact, across health boards, estimated five-year survival rates ranged from 67 per cent to 84 per cent. One possible explanation was differences between health boards in the proportion of patients receiving adjuvant systemic therapy (usually tamoxifen). Analysis clearly showed that the health board of first treatment predicted independently whether or not patients would receive adjuvant systemic treatment.[24]

Figure 6

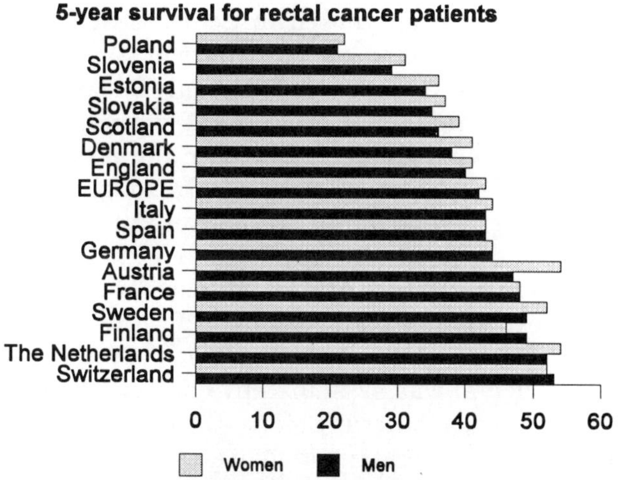

Figure 7

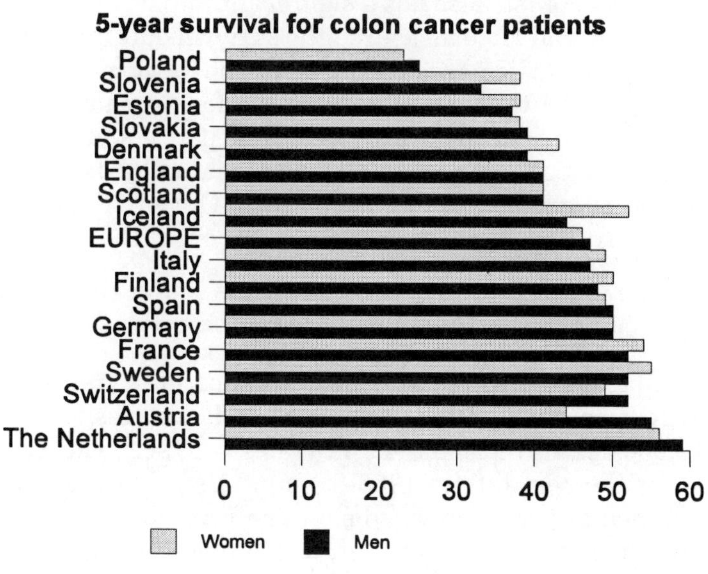

Note: Rates are relative and age-standardised. 1985-1989, Eurocare II

Other studies have also found unexplained variations in diagnosis and treatment. Chouillet and colleagues assessed 334 cases of breast cancer diagnosed in South East England. It is fundamental to effective treatment that the stage of the cancer should be known, but it was recorded in only 24 per cent of cases. Liver and bone scanning and skeletal radiography were carried out as frequently as axillary surgery, when the guidelines advised against the use of such investigations and strongly recommended axillary sampling to determine the stage of the disease.[25]

Sainsbury and colleagues investigated outcomes in 12,861 women treated in Yorkshire and found considerable variations in survival between patients treated by different surgeons. After allowing for case-mix and other variables, 20 per cent of the variation in survival was explained by chemotherapy alone and six per cent by hormone therapy alone. If chemotherapy had been used in 40 per cent of cases (instead of about nine per cent) there would have been a four per cent increase in the five-year survival rate, which would have meant that an additional 500 patients would have been alive after five years.[26]

Access to specialists also has a significant impact on survival. A study by Gillis and Hole measured the survival outcome of care by specialist surgeons in breast cancer in the west of Scotland. [27] This study found that, after adjustment for prognostic factors, five- and ten-year survival rates were nine per cent and eight per cent higher respectively among women treated by breast cancer specialists as opposed to non-specialists. Out of 3,786 patients studied, only 918 were seen by a surgeon with a 'specialist interest'.[28]

Colorectal Cancer

Colorectal cancer is the second most common fatal malignancy in both sexes combined, after lung cancer.[29] It was responsible for over 15,000 deaths in England and Wales in 1996.[30] The Eurocare II study of the period from 1985-89 found that five-year survival for both men and women was below the European average. For England the rate was 41 per cent, which placed it twelfth out of 17. Rates in the most successful countries were substantially higher. The five-year survival rate in the Netherlands was 59 per cent for men and 56 per cent for women. In France the rate was 52 per cent for men and 54 per cent for women.[31]

Ovarian Cancer

Ovarian cancer is the fourth most common cause of death from cancer amongst females, with an overall five-year relative survival rate of just under 30 per cent. There are 6,000 new cases and some 4,000 deaths from ovarian cancer a year.[32]

One study audited seven district health authorities in the South East Thames region covering 118 newly-diagnosed cases of ovarian cancer. Clinical guidelines were agreed before the study began and their implementation was then audited. The guidelines were based on consensus statements and were very similar to guidelines in use in the US and elsewhere in the UK. Both investigation and management of ovarian cancer varied significantly between hospitals. Only 53 per cent of patients received the recommended diagnostic procedures, and the inappropriate investigation may explain the inadequacy of subsequent treatment. Overall, only 43 per cent of patients were judged to have been the subject of 'appropriate clinical investigation and management'. At Stage I, 72 per cent were judged to have been 'inappropriately managed', at Stage II, 47 per cent and at Stage III, 54 per cent were considered to have been 'inappropriately managed', when their treatment was judged against internationally accepted guidelines.[33]

Another retrospective review of patients in Manchester found that fewer than half the patients underwent the generally accepted surgical procedure.[34] The actual conduct of consultants was compared with the 'optimal management' defined in accepted consensus statements.[35] The study found that in North West England many consultants were operating on a few patients each, at the expense of patient survival. The recommended practice was for patients to be treated by specialist teams with the necessary combined expertise and not by individual consultants who lacked the required experience and knowledge. However, in one subset of 76 patients, only 32 received the recommended treatment of hysterectomy, bilateral salpingo-oophorectomy and infracolic omentectomy.[36]

The CancerBACUP survey of ovarian cancer treatment similarly found that various international as well as national guidelines were not being followed. The use of platinum/paclitaxel (Taxol) combination therapy for ovarian cancer had been recommended by the Joint Council for Clinical Oncology (a joint body representing the Royal College of Physicians and the Royal College of Radiologists) and endorsed by the Department of Health's Standing Medical Advisory Committee. First-line use of platinum and Taxol had resulted in more than 70 per cent remission rates and an additional year of life on average.[37]

Figure 8

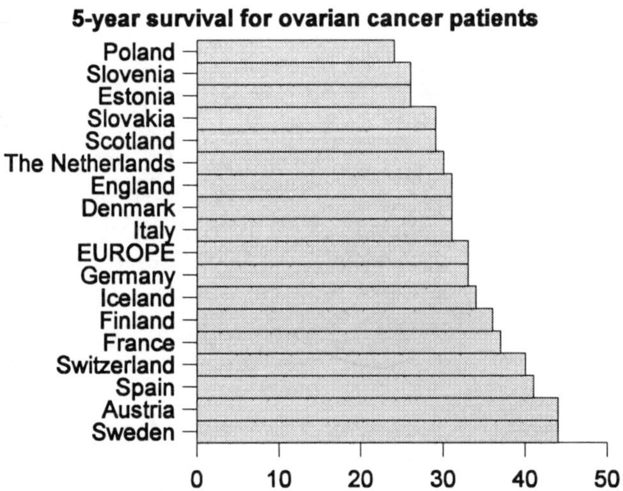

Note: Rates are age standardised and relative. 1985-1989 Eurocare II

In the CancerBACUP survey, individuals who were responsible for commissioning services for around half the nation's population working in 60 NHS authorities and boards were interviewed in the summer of 1998. Less than one-fifth of NHS authorities and boards were able to ensure that suitable ovarian cancer patients received the recommended platinum/paclitaxel treatment. In fact, in many localities there were no patients receiving this treatment from the NHS. The cause was almost entirely financial, because almost all the directors of public health and consultants approached by the survey team were aware of the effectiveness of platinum/paclitaxel treatment. One lead purchaser in southern England commented: 'we recognise that we have got to respond ... The advantages are too great to ignore. But at the same time there are cost questions, and people have got to think through the implications.'[38]

In 1996 the Enfield-Haringey Health Authority sent out a letter to two trusts with which it had contracts urging them to cut back on patients receiving the taxanes, Taxotere (docetaxel) for ovarian and breast cancer and Taxol (paclitaxel). The authority, £1.7m in debt, declared it was taking the action because it had run out of money for treatment using the drugs.[39]

Chemotherapy for cancer has been found to be effective in clinical trials, but not only is it withheld from patients, there are also difficulties in funding further vital research. R.E. Hawkins, Clinical Editor of the *British Journal of Cancer* and Director of Medical Oncology at the Christie CRC Research Centre, has reported that some trials of potentially useful drugs have been delayed because of a lack of funding. The ICON3 trial, for example, was delayed because local purchasers refused to fund the drug costs.

Conclusions

Some of the disparities described were due to bad or inconsistent clinical practice, but the underlying difficulty was the lack of finance.

It is now accepted that adjuvant chemotherapy improves survival and that palliative chemotherapy improves the quality of life for sufferers of advanced cancers. However, in a letter to the *British Medical Journal* in September 1997 eleven doctors representing the Association of Cancer Physicians pointed out that the reallocation of NHS funding to primary care had been the cause of massive problems for cancer units and centres and that cytotoxic therapy had often been the main target for budget reductions. Their use had, in effect, not been funded in many regions. The eleven doctors compared the cost of cytotoxic chemotherapy with other drugs. The total budget for cytotoxic drugs was about £58m compared with the £250m spent on the single ulcer-healing drug omeprazole.[40] The authors quote information from Intercontinental Medical Statistics, for the year ending September 1996, when about £1,038 million was spent on gastrointestinal drugs, £848 million on cardiovascular medicines, £282 million on dermatological treatments and only £167 million on cancer drugs.

The situation had become bad enough by October 1999 for the Secretary of State for Health, Alan Milburn, to announce a new ten-year initiative to improve cancer care. Professor Mike Richards was appointed the National Cancer Director to lead the programme and Mr Milburn declared that he had asked the National Institute for Clinical Excellence to draft early guidance on the use of the taxanes, to 'end the postcode lottery of care', as his press release puts it.[41] He also announced an 'additional' £80 million for cancer services, but when questioned by journalists it turned out that the £80 million was coming out of a sum already allocated for NHS improvements and which had already been announced.[42] Such measures give the impression of action but, in reality, fall a long way short of what is required.

3

Conclusions

The main findings can be summarised as follows. The UK has a poor record of preventing death from diseases of the circulatory system. After allowing for the different age structure of each country in the European Union, the UK death rate from circulatory diseases for persons aged under 65 was ranked thirteenth out of the 15 countries studied.

The two main diseases of the circulatory system are coronary heart disease and stroke. Coronary heart disease is the biggest single cause of premature death, killing 28 per cent of men and 17 per cent of women in 1996. High blood pressure is one of the main risk factors and a successful service would pride itself on effective treatment. However, in 1997 under half of people with high blood pressure were being treated successfully (42 per cent were receiving effective treatment, 21 per cent were being treated inadequately, and 37 per cent were not being treated at all).

Stroke is the third biggest killer and the biggest cause of severe disability. There has been solid evidence for some time that care of stroke patients in a specialised stroke unit reduces mortality by 25 per cent. An effective health service would pride itself on providing for stroke patients in this manner. However, in 1998 only one-third of NHS consultants said that their patients were usually managed by a stroke unit team or in a stroke unit.

It is also difficult to take any pride in the UK's record in cancer care. The best evidence comes from the 17-nation Eurocare study which compares one-year and five-year survival rates for the main cancers. It found that England and Scotland had the lowest one-year survival rates for lung cancer. The five-year survival rate was little better, with England ranking 12 out of 17, above Scotland, Estonia, Denmark, Poland and Slovenia.

For breast cancer (15,000 deaths) England's one-year survival was ranked tenth out of 17 and Scotland's twelfth out of 17, above Austria, Estonia, Poland and Slovakia. The five-year survival rate in England was eleventh out of 17 and in Scotland twelfth out of 17, above Slovenia, Austria, Estonia, Poland, and Slovakia.

Colorectal cancer is the second largest killer affecting both sexes (15,000 deaths). For cancer of the colon in men the five-year survival rate in Scotland and England was ranked equal eleventh out of 17. For women, Scotland and England were equal twelfth out of 17.

Ovarian cancer is the fourth largest cancer killer. The five-year survival rate for England was eleventh out of 17 and for Scotland thirteenth (see Figure 8).

There is little doubt that rationing is the root cause of these problems. In the early 1990s Britain had fewer radiotherapists per head than Poland and fewer medical oncologists than any country in western Europe.[1] The shortage of specialists reflects the general scarcity of doctors. OECD figures for 1996 show that the UK had 1.7 practising physicians per 1,000 population. Germany had 3.4 per 1,000, France 2.9 and Poland 2.4. The only countries with a lower proportion among the 29 studied by the OECD were Korea (1.2), Mexico (1.2) and Turkey (1.1).[2] However well motivated individual doctors might be, if they are in short supply, the inevitable result is the dilution of care.

Total spending on health care is low by international standards. In 1997 total expenditure on health care in the UK was 6.9 per cent of GDP. The German figure was 10.7 per cent and the French, 9.6 per cent. Of the 29 advanced countries studied by the OECD, only Hungary, Ireland, Korea, Mexico, Poland and Turkey spent less. To match German levels would require an increase of nearly £30 billion per year. Even if we leave out private expenditure on health and compare only government spending, the disparity remains. In 1997 the UK government spent 5.8 per cent of GDP on health care, compared with the German figure of 8.3 per cent. To match the German proportion would require nearly £20 billion a year extra. Gaps of this magnitude cannot be closed by measures such as special improvement funds and efficiency savings.

What should be done? After decades of denial it is now widely accepted that NHS rationing is endemic and has harmful consequences for patients. Would 'more money' be the answer?

This is not the place to go into the complex issues entailed in any search for an alternative to the NHS, but state finance has now been tested in a 50-year pilot scheme which any reasonable and impartial observer would concede has been a failure. We need an urgent public debate about how best to introduce a bigger role for personal payment and insurance without compromising the principle of access for all.

There are countless alternatives available elsewhere in the world and a debate has already begun in the UK. For example, Professor Chris Ham, has advocated an increased role for competing non-profits.[3] Professor John Spiers has advocated the privatisation of hospitals.[4] John Willman, Consumer Industries Editor of the *Financial Times,* has advocated patient charges.[5] And Oliver Morgan of the *Observer* has put the case for increased private finance.[6] We hope that our findings will add a little urgency to the search for a better alternative.

Notes

Introduction

1 For instance, Cooper, L., Coote, A., Davies, A. and Jackson, C., *Voices Off: Tackling the Democratic Deficit in Health*, London: Institute for Public Policy Research, 1995.

2 For example, Professor Alan Maynard at the University of York is a strong defender of this approach. The journal *Effective Health Care* regularly publishes studies of cost-effectiveness.

3 See for example the publications of Professor Alan Williams, University of York.

4 Hunter, D., *Desperately Seeking Solutions*, London: Longman, 1997.

5 Klein, R., Day, P. and Redmayne, S., *Managing Scarcity: Priority Setting and Rationing in the National Health Service*, Buckingham: Open University Press, 1996.

6 Klein *et al.*, *Managing Scarcity,* 1996, p. 123.

7 McKenzie, J. *et al.*, 'Dialysis decision making in Canada, the United Kingdom and the United States', *American Journal of Kidney Diseases,* Vol. 31, No. 1 (January) 1998, pp. 12-18.

8 Roderick, P. *et al.*, 'The provision of renal replacement therapy for adults in England and Wales: recent trends and future directions', *Q J Med*, Vol. 91, 1998, pp. 581-87.

9 Department of Health, *The National Survey of NHS Patients.* <www.doh.gov.uk/public/nhssurvey.htm>

10 The Clinical Standards Advisory Group was established in April 1991, under Section 62 of the NHS and Community Care Act 1990, as an independent source of expert advice to UK health ministers and to the NHS on standards of clinical care for, and access and availability of services to, NHS patients. The Group's members are nominated by the medical, nursing and dental royal colleges and their faculties, the professions allied to medicine, and include the chairman of the Standing Medical Advisory Committee.

11 The Standing Medical Advisory Committee is one of five statutory bodies which advise health ministers in England and Wales on the provision of medical services under the NHS Acts. Members are appointed by ministers following nominations by

professional bodies and include the presidents of all medical royal colleges. Nine standing advisory committees were first established in 1949, but under the NHS (SAC) Order 1981, four SACs were retained with unchanged terms of reference, to advise on the provision of medical, nursing & midwifery, dental, and pharmaceutical services in England and Wales. A fifth SAC, now the Joint Committee for Vaccination and Immunisation Services, was subsequently established. SACs perform their statutory functions in three ways: developing advice (advisory role); commenting on advice developed by others (consultative role); and alerting ministers and the department to issues which are likely to be important in the future (monitoring role).

Chapter 1

1 *Coronary Heart Disease Statistics*, British Heart Foundation, 1998, p. 14.

2 *Coronary Heart Disease Statistics*, 1998, p. 9.

3 *Saving Lives: Our Healthier Nation,* Cm. 4386, London: The Stationery Office, 1999, p. 73. See also Dept of Health, *Coronary Heart Disease: An Epidemiological Overview*, London: HMSO, 1994.

4 *Coronary Heart Disease Statistics*, 1998, p. 14.

5 *The Health of the Nation,* Cm 1523, London: HMSO, 1991, p. 59.

6 *Coronary Heart Disease Statistics*, 1998, pp. 9-10, 19. The figures are for men aged 35-74 and are age-standardised, based on the European Standard Population.

7 *Coronary Heart Disease Statistics*, 1998, p. 34.

8 *Coronary Heart Disease Statistics*, 1998, p. 84.

9 Coronary angioplasty involves inserting a balloon into the obstructed artery and inflating it to tear the inner part of the arterial wall in order to reduce the obstruction. The CABG is a better method of relieving heart pain than angioplasty, but because of the higher risk of death it is more appropriate for high-risk patients. See, for example, NHS Centre for Reviews and Dissemination, 'Management of stable angina', *Effective Health Care*, October 1997, vol. 3, no. 5.

10 *Health of the Nation*, 1991, p. 59.

11 *Coronary Heart Disease Statistics,* 1998, p. 43. Population estimates from *Annual Abstract of Statistics.*

12 Audit Commission, *Dear to Our Hearts*, London: HMSO, 1995, p. 20.

13 American Heart Association <www.americanheart.org> and US Census Bureau.

14 OECD, Health Data 1999 (CD), Paris: OECD.

15 Department of Health, *Saving Lives: Our Healthier Nation*, Cm 4386, London: TSO, July 1999, p. 80.

16 Audit Commission, *Dear to Our Hearts*, London: HMSO, 1995, p. 20.

17 Billing, J.S., Arifi, A.A., Sharples, L.D., Tsui, S.S.L., Nashef, S.A.M., 'Heart surgery in UK patients: planned care or crisis management?' *Lancet*, Vol. 347, 24 February 1996, pp. 540-41.

18 Clinical Standards Advisory Group, *Coronary Artery Bypass Grafting and Coronary Angioplasty. Access to and Availability of Specialist Services,* London: HMSO, 1993.

19 Kee, F., McDonald, P., Kirwan, J.R., Patterson, C.C., Love, A.H.G., 'Urgency and priority for cardiac surgery: a clinical judgement analysis,' *British Medical Journal*, 1998; 316: 925-929 (21 March). See also Macleod, M. *et al.*., 'Geographic, demographic and socioeconomic variations in the investigation and management of coronary heart disease in Scotland', *Heart*, 1999; 81:252-256.

20 Grimley Evans, J., 'This patient or that patient', in Smith, R. (ed.), *Rationing in Action*, London: British Medical Journal, 1993.

21 Underwood, M.J. and Bailey, J.S., 'Should smokers be offered coronary bypass surgery?', *British Medical Journal* 1993; 306: 1047-50 (17 April).

22 *Coronary Heart Disease Statistics,* 1998, p. 73.

23 World Health Organisation and International Society of Hypertension, *1999 WHO/ISH Hypertension Guidelines.*

24 Calcium antagonists also cause blood vessels to dilate, but by a different mechanism.

25 Eccles, M., Freemantle, N. and Mason, J., 'North of England evidence based development project: guideline for angiotensin converting enzyme inhibitors in primary care management of adults with symptomatic heart failure', *British Medical Journal,* 1998;316:1369-1375 (2 May).

26 Eccles *et al.*, 'North of England evidence based development project: guideline for angiotensin converting enzyme inhibitors in primary care management of adults with symptomatic heart failure', *British Medical Journal,* 1998; 316:1369-1375 (2 May).

27 Jones, J., Brown A. and Waugh, N., *SHPIC Report –1998: Heart Failure*, Scotland Health Purchasing Information Centre, 1998.

28 Campbell, N. *et al.*, 'Secondary prevention in coronary heart disease: baseline survey of provision in general practice', *British Medical Journal*,1998; 316:1430-1434 (9 May).

29 McGrae McDermott, M., Feinglass, J., Lee, P., Mehta, S., Schmitt, B., Lefevre, F., Puppala J. and Gheorghiade M., 'Heart failure between 1986 and 1994: temporal trends in drug-prescribing practices, hospital readmissions, and survival at an academic medical center', *American Heart Journal,*, 134(5): 901-909, 1997.

30 Jones, Brown and Waugh, *SHPIC Report–1998: Heart Failure.*

31 Francis, C.M. *et al.*, 'Open access echocardiography in management of heart failure in the community', *British Medical Journal*, 1995; 310:634-6 (11 March).

32 Jones, Brown and Waugh, *SHPIC Report - 1998: Heart Failure.*

33 Eccles *et al.*, 'North of England evidence based development project: guideline for angiotensin converting enzyme inhibitors in primary care management of adults with symptomatic heart failure', *British Medical Journal,* 1998;316:1369-1375 (2 May). See also Clarke, K.W. *et al.*, 'Evidence of inadequate investigation and treatment of patients with heart failure', *British Heart Journal*, 1994; 71: 584-87.

34 Eccles *et al.*, 'North of England evidence based development project: guideline for angiotensin converting enzyme inhibitors in primary care management of adults with symptomatic heart failure', *British Medical Journal,* 1998;316:1369-1375 (2 May).

35 *Coronary Heart Disease Statistics*, 1998, p. 73.

36 Department of Health, *Saving Lives: Our Healthier Nation*, Cm 4386, London: TSO, July 1999, p. 77.

37 *Coronary Heart Disease Statistics*, 1998, p. 77.

38 NHS Centre for Reviews and Dissemination, 'Cholesterol and coronary heart disease: screening and treatment', *Effective Health Care,* Vol. 4, No. 1, February 1998.

39 'Randomised trial of cholesterol lowering in 4,444 patients with coronary heart disease: the Scandinavian Simvastatin Survival Study (4S)', *Lancet*, 1994 (November 19); 344(8934):1383-9.

40 Baxter, C., Jones, R. and Corr, L., 'Time trend analysis and variations in prescribing lipid lowering drugs in general practice,' *British Medical Journal*, 1998; 317:1134-1135 (24 Oct).

41 NHS Centre for Reviews and Dissemination, 'Cholesterol and coronary heart disease: screening and treatment', *Effective Health Care,* Vol. 4, No. 1, February 1998.

42 Department of Health, Statistics division 1E, 'Prescription cost analysis system in: cholesterol and coronary heart disease: screening and treatment', *Effective Health Care,* Vol. 4, No. 1, February 1998.

43 NHS Centre for Reviews and Dissemination, 'Cholesterol and coronary heart disease: screening and treatment', *Effective Health Care,* Vol. 4, No. 1, February 1998.

44 ASPIRE Steering Group, 'A British Cardiac Society survey of the potential for the secondary prevention of heart disease', *Heart*, 1996; 75: 334-342.

45 Baxter, C., Jones, R. and Corr, L., 'Time trend analysis and variations in prescribing lipid lowering drugs in general practice,' *British Medical Journal*,1998; 317:1134-1135 (24 Oct).

46 Campbell, N. *et al.*, 'Secondary prevention in coronary heart disease: baseline survey of provision in general practice', *British Medical Journal*, 1998; 316:1430-1434 (9 May).

47 Standing Medical Advisory Committee, *The Use of Statins,* Department of Health, 1997.

48 NHS Centre for Reviews and Dissemination, 'Cholesterol and coronary heart disease: screening and treatment', *Effective Health Care,* Vol. 4, No. 1, February 1998.

49 Freemantle, N., Barbour, R., Johnson, R., Marchment, M., Kennedy, A., 'The use of statins: a case of misleading priorities?' *British Medical Journal*,1997; 315:826-828 (4 Oct).

50 Audit Commission, *Improving Value For Money in the NHS: A Compendium of Good Practice from Audit Commission Reports*, London: Audit Commission, August 1999, p. 57.

51 Audit Commission, *Dear to Our Hearts*, 1995, p. 55.

52 Crail, M., 'Never mind the quality...', *Health Service Journal*, Vol. 1, April 1999, pp. 12-13.

53 NHS Centre for Reviews and Dissemination, 'Cardiac rehabilitation,' *Effective Health Care*, Vol. 4, No. 4, August 1998.

54 *Stroke Care: A Matter of Chance*, London: The Stroke Association, 1999. See also Dept of Health, *Stroke: An Epidemiological Overview*, London: HMSO, 1994.

55 *Stroke Care: Reducing the Burden of Disease*, London: The Stroke Association, 1998, p. 6.

56 Geddes, J. *et al.*, 'Prevalence of self-reported stroke in a population in northern England', *Journal of Epidemiology and Community Health,* 1996; 50: 140-143.

57 *Stroke Care: Reducing the Burden of Disease*, 1998, p. 12.

58 *Stroke Care: A Matter of Chance,* 1999.

59 Kalra, L., 'The influence of stroke unit rehabilitation on the functional recovery from stroke', *Stroke*, 1994; 25: 821-25.

60 Langhorne, P., Williams, B., Gilchrist, W. and Howie, K., 'Do stroke units save lives?', *Lancet* 1993; 342: 395-98 (14 August).

61 Stroke Unit Trialists' Collaboration, 'Collaborative systematic review of the randomised trials of organised inpatient (stroke unit) care after stroke', *British Medical Journal,* 1997;314:1151 (19 April).

62 *Stroke Care: A Matter of Chance*, 1999, p. 10.

63 *Stroke Care: A Matter of Chance*, 1999, p. 11.

64 *Stroke Care: A Matter of Chance*, 1999.

65 *Stroke Care: A Matter of Chance*, 1999, pp. 12-13.

66 *Stroke Care: A Matter of Chance*, 1999, pp. 15, 30.

67 *Stroke Care: A Matter of Chance*, 1999, pp. 17-18.

Chapter 2

1 *Saving Lives: Our Healthier Nation,* Cm. 4386, London: TSO, July 1999, p. 61.

2 *Saving Lives: Our Healthier Nation,* 1999, p. 62.

3 Berrino, F., Gatta, G., Chessa, E., Valenie, F. and Capocaccia, R., Introduction: the EUROCARE II Study, *European Journal of Cancer*, Vol. 34, No. 14, 1998, pp. 2139-53.

4 Gatta, J. *et al.*, 'Survival of colorectal cancer patients in Europe during the period 1978-1989', *European Journal of Cancer*, Vol. 34, No. 14, 1998, pp. 2176-83.

5 Janssen-Heijnen, M. *et al.*, 'Variation in survival of patients with lung cancer in Europe, 1985-1989', *European Journal of Cancer,* Vol. 34, No. 14, 1998, pp. 2191-96.

6 Quinn, M. *et al.*, 'Variations in survival from breast cancer in Europe by age and country, 1978-1989', *European Journal of Cancer,* Vol. 34, No. 14, 1998, pp. 2204-11.

7 Chief Medical Officer's Expert Advisory Group on Cancer, *Policy Framework for Commissioning Cancer Services,* London: Department of Health, 1995.

8 Sikora, K., 'Rationing cancer care' in Spiers, J. (ed.), *The Realities of Rationing*, London: IEA, 1999, p. 136.

9 Husband, D.J., 'Malignant spinal cord compression: prospective study of delays in referral and treatment', *British Medical Journal,* 1998; 317:18-21 (4 July).

10 Richards, M.A. and Parrott, C., 'Tertiary cancer services in Britain: benchmarking study of activity and facilities at 12 specialist centres,' *British Medical Journal,* 1996; 313: 347 - 349 (10 August).

11 Richards and Parrott, 'Tertiary cancer services in Britain: benchmarking study of activity and facilities at 12 specialist centres,' *British Medical Journal,* 1996; 313: 347 - 349 (10 August).

12 Sikora, 'Rationing cancer care' in *The Realities of Rationing*, 1999, pp. 134-35.

13 Sikora, K., 'Cancer survival in Britain', *British Medical Journal*, 1999; 319:461-462 (21 August).

14 Sikora, 'Rationing cancer care' in *The Realities of Rationing*, 1999, p. 127.

15 Laroche, C., Wells, F., Coulden, R., Stewart, S., Goddard, M., Lowry, E., Price, A. and Gilligan, D., 'Improving surgical resection rate in lung cancer', *Thorax*, 1998 June, 53:6, 445-9.

16 Janssen-Heijnen, M. et al., 'Variation in survival of patients with lung cancer in Europe, 1985-1989', *European Journal of Cancer,* Vol. 34, No. 14, pp. 2191-96, 1998.

17 Pickles, H., 'Treating lung cancer in the NHS market', *British Medical Journal*, 1997; 315: 1548-1549 (6 December).

18 Sant, M., Capocaccia, R., Verdecchia, A., Esteve, J., Gatta, G., Micheli, A., Coleman, M.P., Berrino, F. and the EUROCARE Working Group, 'Survival of women with breast cancer in Europe - variation with age, year of diagnosis and country', *Int J Cancer*: 77, 679-683 (1998).

19 Quinn, M. *et al.*, 'Variations in survival from breast cancer in Europe by age and country, 1978-1989', *European Journal of Cancer,* Vol 34, No. 14, pp. 2204-2211, 1998.

20 Sant *et al.*, 'Survival of women with breast cancer in Europe: variation with age, year of diagnosis and country', *Int J Cancer*: 77, 679-683 (1998).

21 Richards, M., Sainsbury, R. and Kerr, D., 'Inequalities in breast cancer care and outcome', *British Journal of Cancer,* 1997, 76:5, 634-8.

22 Richards, Sainsbury and Kerr, 'Inequalities in breast cancer care and outcome', *British Journal of Cancer,* 1997, 76:5, 634-5.

23 Richards, M.A. *et al.*, 'Variations in the management and survival of women under 50 years with breast cancer in the South East Thames region', *British Journal of Cancer*, 1996, 73, 751-757.

24 Twelves, C.J., Thomson, C.S., Gould, A., Dewar, J.A., for the Scottish Breast Cancer Focus Group and the Scottish Cancer Therapy Network, 'Variation in the survival of women with breast cancer in Scotland', *British Journal of Cancer*, 1998, 78:5, 566-571.

25 Chouillet, A.M., Bell, C.M. and Hiscox, J.G., 'Management of breast cancer in southeast England', *British Medical Journal* 1994; 308: 168-171 (15 January).

26 Sainsbury, R., Haward, B., Rider, L., Johnston, C. and Round, C., 'Influence of clinician workload and patterns of treatment on survival from breast cancer', *Lancet* 1995; 345 (8960): 1265-70 (May 20).

27 Gillis, C.R. and Hole, D.J., 'Survival outcome of care by specialist surgeons in breast cancer: a study of 3786 patients in the west of Scotland,' *BMJ* 1996; 312:145-148 (20 January).

28 Gillis and Hole, 'Survival outcome of care by specialist surgeons in breast cancer: a study of 3786 patients in the west of Scotland,' *BMJ* 1996; 312:145-148 (20 January). See also Gillis' reply to critics in 'Authors' reply', *BMJ* 1996; 313:495 (24 August).

29 Dunlop, M.G., 'Science, medicine and the future: Colorectal Cancer,' *BMJ* 1997; 314:1882 (28 June).

30 NHS Centre for Reviews and Dissemination, 'The management of colorectal cancer', *Effective Health Care*, December 1997 Vol. 3, No. 6. (68% cancer of the colon; 32% cancer of the rectum.)

31 Gatta, J. *et al.*, 'Survival of colorectal cancer patients in Europe during the period 1978-1989', *European Journal of Cancer*, Vol. 34, No. 14, pp. 2176-83, 1998.

32 Taylor, D. and Mossman, J., *Living with Ovarian Cancer: A CancerBACUP survey*, London: CancerBACUP, 1999.

33 Wolfe, C.D.A., Tilling, K., Raju, K.S., 'Management and survival of ovarian cancer patients in South East England,' *European Journal of Cancer,* Vol. 33, No. 11, Oct 1997 pp. 1835-1840.

34 Sengupta, P.S., Jayson, G.C., Slade, R.J., Eardley, A. and Radford, J.A., 'An audit of primary surgical treatment for women with ovarian cancer referred to a cancer centre,' *British Journal of Cancer,* Vol. 80, No. 3/4, May 1999, pp. 444-47.

35 Scott, J.S. (1991) *Management of ovarian cancer: current clinical practices.* (Report of a working group), London: SMAC, 1991. See also Allen, D.G. *et al.*, 'Advanced epithelial ovarian cancer: 1993 consensus statements', *Ann Oncol* 4 (Suppl 4):S83-S88, 1993.

36 Sengupta, Jayson, Slade, Eardley and Radford, 'An audit of primary surgical treatment for women with ovarian cancer referred to a cancer centre', *British Journal of Cancer*, Vol. 80, No 3/4, May 1999, pp. 444-47.

37 Taylor and Mossman, *Living with Ovarian Cancer: A CancerBACUP Care Survey*, 1999.

38 Taylor and Mossman, *Living with Ovarian Cancer: A CancerBACUP Care Survey*, 1999, p. 12.

39 Halle, M., 'Cancer treatments rationed by authority,' *BMJ* 1996; 313:774 (28 September).

40 Leonard, R.C.F., Smith, I.E., Coleman, R.E., Malpas, J.S., Nicolson, M., Cassidy, J., Jones, A., McIllmurray, M.B., Stuart, N.S.A., Woll, P.J. and Whithouse, J.M.A., Members of the executive committee of the Association of Cancer Physicians, 'More money is needed to care for patients with cancer', *BMJ* 1997; 315:811-812 (27 September).

41 Department of Health, press release 1999/0631.

42 *The Times*, 26 October 1999.

Conclusions

1 Sikora, K., 'Cancer survival in Britain', *British Medical Journal*, 1999; 319:461-462 (21 August).

2 *OECD Health Data 99 (CD).*

3 Ham, C., *Public, Private or Community: What Next for the NHS?*, London: Demos, 1996.

4 Spiers, J. (ed.), *The Realities of Rationing: 'Priority Setting' in the NHS*, London: IEA, 1999.

5 Willman, J., *A Better State of Health*, London: Social Market Foundation, 1998.

6 Morgan, O., *A Cue for Change: Global Comparisons in Health Care*, London: Social Market Foundation, 1999.

IEA Health and Welfare Unit

Independence

The Health and Welfare Unit is part of the Institute of Economic Affairs, a registered educational charity (No. 235351) founded in 1955. Like the IEA, the Health and Welfare Unit is financed from a variety of private sources to avoid over-reliance on any single or small group of donors.

All IEA publications are independently refereed and referees' comments are passed on anonymously to authors. The IEA gratefully acknowledges the contributions made to its educational work by the eminent scholars who act as referees.

All the Institute's publications seek to further its objective of promoting the advancement of learning, by research into economic and political science, by education of the public therein, and by the dissemination of ideas, research and the results of research in these subjects. The views expressed are those of the authors, not of the IEA, which has no corporate view.